The Affordable Vegetarian Salad Cooking Guide

Easy And Affordable Vegetarian Salad
Recipes For Everyone

Lucas Pearson

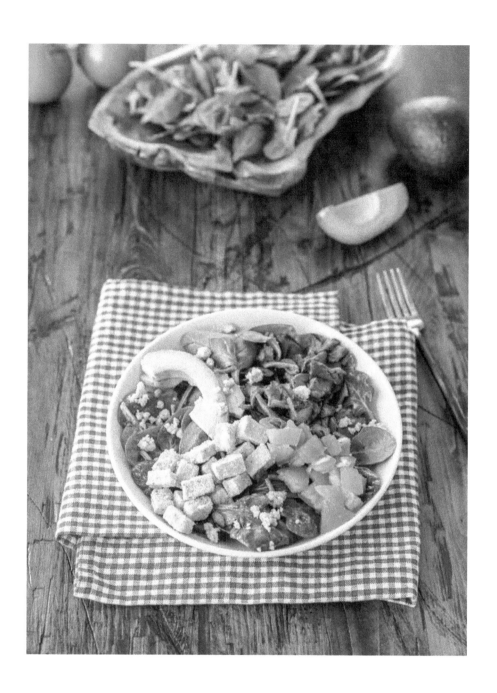

Table of contents

5

Endive and Enoki Mushroom with Mozzarella Cheese Salad

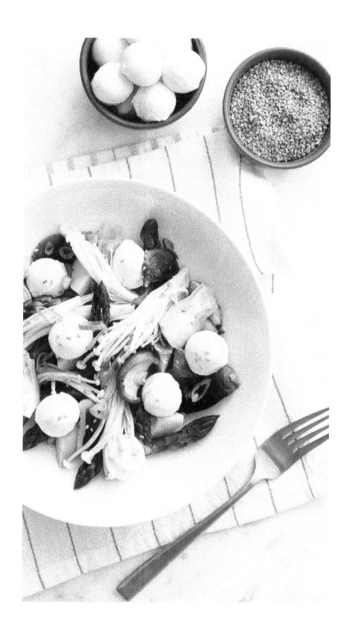

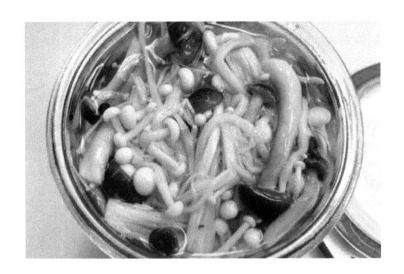

Ingredients:

- 1 bunch Endive, rinsed and drained
- 15 Enoki Mushrooms, thinly sliced
- 1/4 white onion, peeled, halved lengthwise, and thinly sliced
- 1 large cucumber, halved lengthwise and thinly sliced
- 5 ounces mozarella cheese, shredded

<u>Dressing</u>

- ¼ cup extra-virgin olive oil
- 2 splashes white wine vinegar
- Coarse salt and black pepper

Directions:

Combine all of the dressing ingredients. Toss with the rest of the ingredients and combine well.

Spinach and Heirloom Tomato Salad

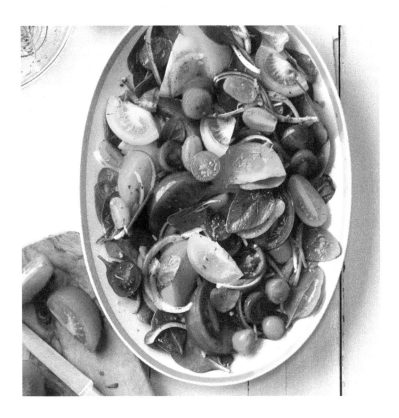

Ingredients:

- 1 bunch Spinach, rinsed and drained

- 3 Heirloom tomatoes, halved lengthwise, seeded, and thinly sliced

- 1/4 white onion, peeled, halved lengthwise, and thinly sliced

- 1 large cucumber, halved lengthwise and thinly sliced

<u>Dressing</u>

- ¼ cup extra-virgin olive oil

- 2 tbsp. apple cider vinegar

- Coarse salt and black pepper

Directions:

Combine all of the dressing ingredients. Toss with the rest of the ingredients and combine well.

Mesclun and Enoki Mushroom Salad

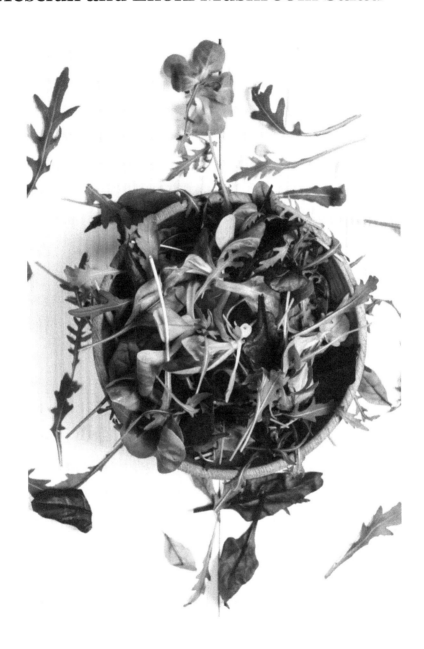

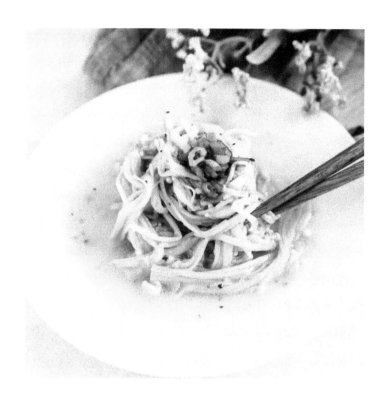

Ingredients:

- 1 bunch Meslcun, rinsed and drained

- 15 Enoki Mushrooms, thinly sliced

- 1/4 white onion, peeled, halved lengthwise, and thinly sliced

- 1 large cucumber, halved lengthwise and thinly sliced

- 5 ounces ricotta cheese

Dressing

- ¼ cup extra-virgin olive oil

- 2 splashes white wine vinegar

- Coarse salt and black pepper

Directions:

Combine all of the dressing ingredients. Toss with the rest of the ingredients and combine well.

Kale Spinach and Zucchini with Cream Cheese Salad

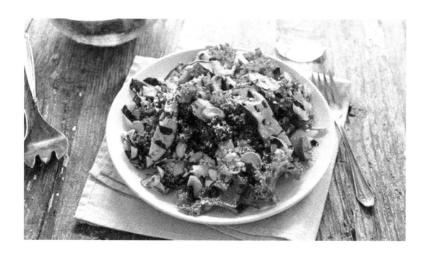

Ingredients:

- 1 bunch Kale, rinsed and drained

- 1 bunch Spinach, rinsed and drained

- 1/4 white onion, peeled, halved lengthwise, and thinly sliced

- 1 large Zucchini halved lengthwise ,thinly sliced and blanched

- 5 ounces cream cheese

Dressing

- ¼ cup extra-virgin olive oil

- 2 splashes white wine vinegar

- Coarse salt and black pepper

Directions:

Combine all of the dressing ingredients. Toss with the rest of the ingredients and combine well.

Kale and Artichoke Salad

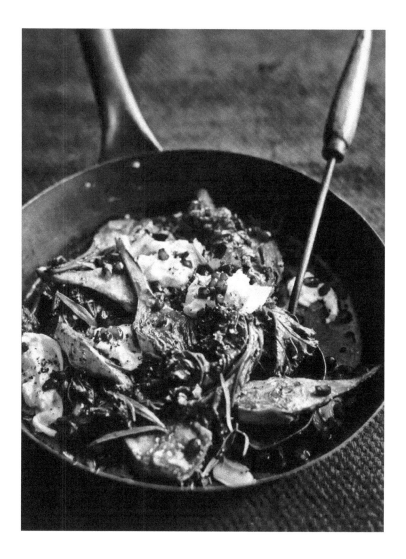

Ingredients:

- 1 bunch Kale, rinsed and drained

- 1 Artichoke, rinsed and drained

- 1 large cucumber, halved lengthwise and thinly sliced

- 5 ounces mozarella cheese, shredded

<u>Dressing</u>

- ¼ cup extra-virgin olive oil

- 2 splashes white wine vinegar

- Coarse salt and black pepper

Directions:

Combine all of the dressing ingredients. Toss with the rest of the ingredients and combine well.

Kale and Romaine Lettuce Salad

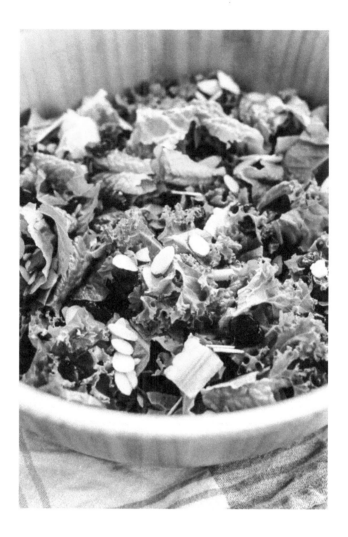

Ingredients:

- 1 bunch Kale, rinsed and drained

- 1 bunch Romaine Lettuce, rinsed and drained

- 1/4 white onion, peeled, halved lengthwise, and thinly sliced

- 1 large cucumber, halved lengthwise and thinly sliced

- 5 ounces cream cheese, crumbled

Dressing

- ¼ cup extra-virgin olive oil

- 2 tbsp. apple cider vinegar

- Coarse salt and black pepper

Directions:

Combine all of the dressing ingredients. Toss with the rest of the ingredients and combine well.

Iceberg Lettuce and Endive Salad

Ingredients:

- 1 bunch Iceberg Lettuce, rinsed and drained
- 1 bunch Endive, rinsed and drained
- 5 medium plum tomatoes, halved lengthwise, seeded, and thinly sliced
- 1/4 white onion, peeled, halved lengthwise, and thinly sliced
- 1 large cucumber, halved lengthwise and thinly sliced

Dressing

- ¼ cup extra-virgin olive oil
- 2 splashes white wine vinegar
- Coarse salt and black pepper

Directions:

Combine all of the dressing ingredients. Toss with the rest of the ingredients and combine well.

Kale and Spinach with Parmesan Cheese Salad

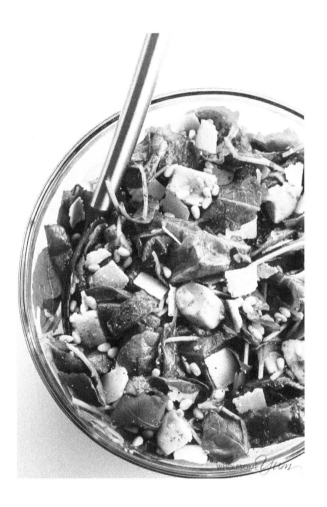

Ingredients:

- 1 bunch Kale, rinsed and drained

- 1 bunch Spinach, rinsed and drained

- 15 Enoki Mushrooms, thinly sliced
- 1/4 white onion, peeled, halved lengthwise, and thinly sliced
- 1 large cucumber, halved lengthwise and thinly sliced
- 5 ounces parmesan cheese, shredded

Dressing

- ¼ cup extra-virgin olive oil
- 2 splashes white wine vinegar
- Coarse salt and black pepper

Directions:

Combine all of the dressing ingredients. Toss with the rest of the ingredients and combine well

Corn and Plum Tomato with Cottage Cheese Salad

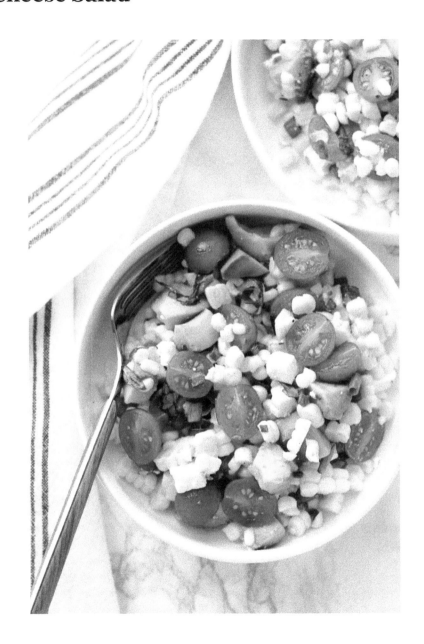

Ingredients:

- 1 cup baby corn (canned), drained
- 5 medium plum tomatoes, halved lengthwise, seeded, and thinly sliced
- 1/4 white onion, peeled, halved lengthwise, and thinly sliced
- 1 large Zucchini halved lengthwise ,thinly sliced and blanched
- 5 ounces cottage cheese, crumbled

Dressing

- ¼ cup extra-virgin olive oil
- 2 splashes white wine vinegar
- Coarse salt and black pepper

Directions:

Combine all of the dressing ingredients. Toss with the rest of the ingredients and combine well.

Boston Lettuce and Baby Corn Salad

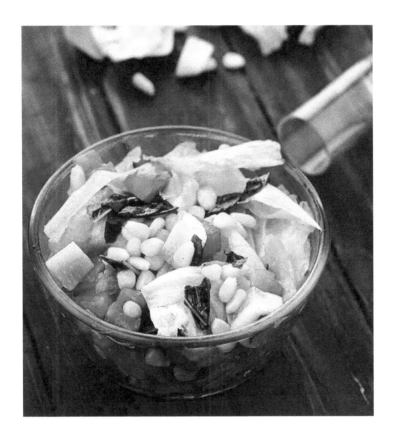

Ingredients:

- 1 bunch Boston Lettuce, rinsed and drained

- 1 cup baby corn (canned), drained

- 1 large cucumber, halved lengthwise and thinly sliced

- 5 ounces monterey jack cheese, shredded

Dressing

- ¼ cup extra-virgin olive oil

- 2 splashes white wine vinegar

- Coarse salt and black pepper

Directions:

Combine all of the dressing ingredients. Toss with the rest of the ingredients and combine well.

Broccoli and Tomatillo Salad

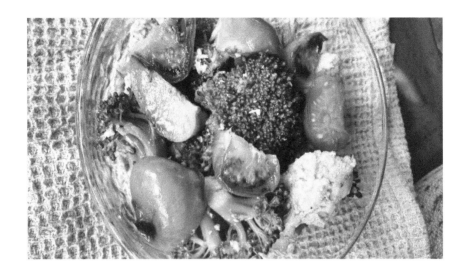

Ingredients:

- 9 broccoli florets, blanched and drained

- 10 Tomatillos, halved lengthwise, seeded, and thinly sliced

- 1/4 white onion, peeled, halved lengthwise, and thinly sliced

- 1 large cucumber, halved lengthwise and thinly sliced

- 5 ounces gouda cheese, shredded

Dressing

- ¼ cup extra-virgin olive oil

- 2 splashes white wine vinegar

- Coarse salt and black pepper

Directions:

Combine all of the dressing ingredients. Toss with the rest of the ingredients and combine well.

Kale and Cauliflower Salad

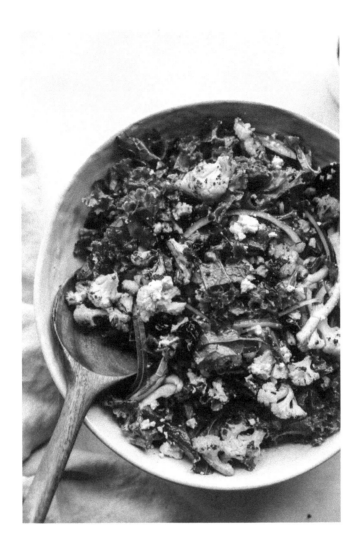

Ingredients:

- 1 bunch Kale, rinsed and drained
- 9 cauliflower florets, blanched and drained

- 1 large Zucchini halved lengthwise, thinly sliced and blanched

- 5 ounces pepperjack cheese, shredded

Dressing

- ¼ cup extra-virgin olive oil

- 2 splashes white wine vinegar

- Coarse salt and black pepper

Directions:

Combine all of the dressing ingredients. Toss with the rest of the ingredients and combine well.

Endives Spinach & Broccoli Salad

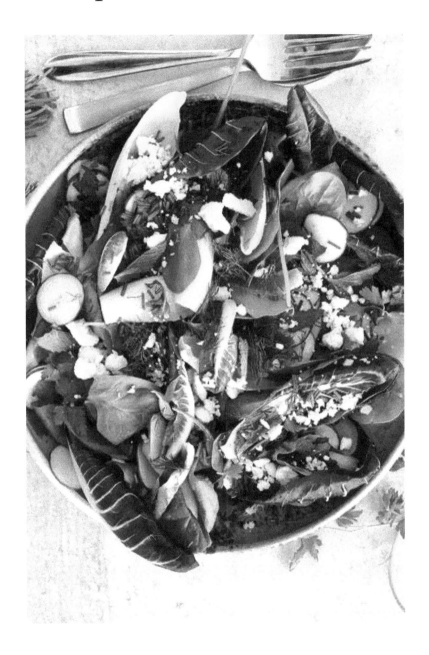

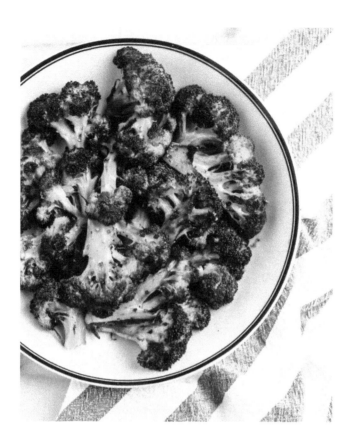

Ingredients:

- 1 bunch Endives, rinsed and drained

- 8 broccoli florets, blanched and drained

- 1 bunch Spinach, rinsed and drained

- 5 ounces cottage cheese, crumbled

Dressing

- ¼ cup extra-virgin olive oil

- 2 splashes white wine vinegar

- Coarse salt and black pepper

Directions:

Combine all of the dressing ingredients. Toss with the rest of the ingredients and combine well.

Baby Corn and Endive Salad

Ingredients:

- 1 cup baby corn (canned), drained
- 1 bunch Collard Greens, rinsed and drained
- 1 Artichoke, rinsed and drained
- 5 ounces pecorino romano cheese, shredded
- 1 ounces cream cheese, crumbled

Dressing

- ¼ cup extra-virgin olive oil
- 2 tbsp. apple cider vinegar
- Coarse salt and black pepper

Directions:

Combine all of the dressing ingredients. Toss with the rest of the ingredients and combine well.

Tomatillo and Baby Corn Salad

Ingredients:

- 10 Tomatillos, halved lengthwise, seeded, and thinly sliced
- 1 cup baby corn (canned), drained
- 1 bunch Endive, rinsed and drained
- 1 Artichoke, rinsed and drained
- 1 ounces monterey jack cheese, shredded
- 5 ounces cheddar cheese, shredded

Dressing

- ¼ cup extra-virgin olive oil
- 2 splashes white wine vinegar
- Coarse salt and black pepper

Directions:

Combine all of the dressing ingredients. Toss with the rest of the ingredients and combine well.

Heirloom Tomato Endive and Artichoke Salad

Ingredients:

- 3 Heirloom tomatoes, halved lengthwise, seeded, and thinly sliced
- 1 bunch Endive, rinsed and drained
- 1 Artichoke, rinsed and drained
- 1 bunch Kale, rinsed and drained

Dressing

- ¼ cup extra-virgin olive oil
- 2 splashes white wine vinegar
- Coarse salt and black pepper

Directions:

Combine all of the dressing ingredients. Toss with the rest of the ingredients and combine well.

Collard Greens Plum Tomatoes and Onion Salad

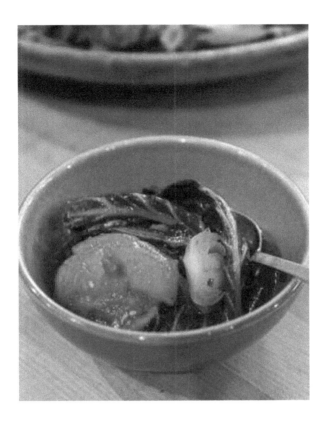

Ingredients:

- 1 bunch of collard greens, rinsed and drained

- 5 medium plum tomatoes, halved lengthwise, seeded, and thinly sliced

- 1/4 white onion, peeled, halved lengthwise, and thinly sliced

- 1 large cucumber, halved lengthwise and thinly sliced

- 5 ounces feta cheese, crumbled

Dressing

- ¼ cup extra-virgin olive oil

- 2 splashes white wine vinegar

- Coarse salt and black pepper

Directions:

Combine all of the dressing ingredients. Toss with the rest of the ingredients and combine well.

Mangoes tomatoes and Cucumber Salad

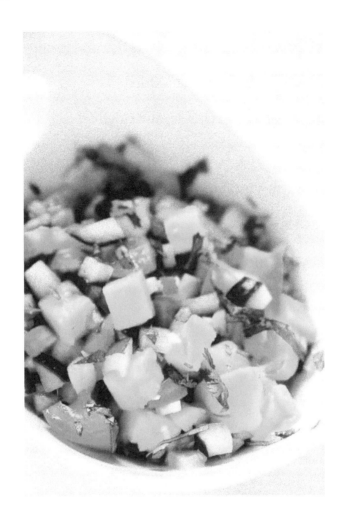

Ingredients:

- 1 cup of cubed mangoes

- 5 medium plum tomatoes, halved lengthwise, seeded, and thinly sliced

- 1/4 white onion, peeled, halved lengthwise, and thinly sliced

- 1 large cucumber, halved lengthwise and thinly sliced

- 3 ounces gouda cheese, shredded

- 3 ounces parmesan cheese, shredded

Dressing

- ¼ cup extra-virgin olive oil

- 2 splashes white wine vinegar

- Coarse salt and black pepper

Directions:

Combine all of the dressing ingredients. Toss with the rest of the ingredients and combine well.

Black Grapes Tomatillo and White Onion

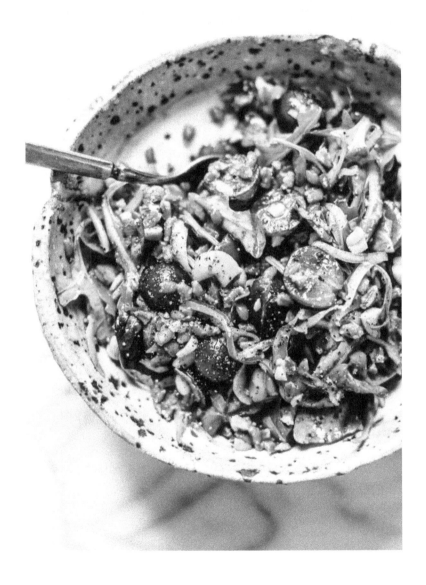

Ingredients:

- 12 pcs. black grapes
- 10 Tomatillos, halved lengthwise, seeded, and thinly sliced
- 1/4 white onion, peeled, halved lengthwise, and thinly sliced
- 1 large cucumber, halved lengthwise and thinly sliced
- 3 ounces pepperjack cheese, shredded
- 3 ounces mozarella cheese, shredded

Dressing

- ¼ cup extra-virgin olive oil
- 2 splashes white wine vinegar
- Coarse salt and black pepper

Directions:

Combine all of the dressing ingredients. Toss with the rest of the ingredients and combine well.

Red Cabbage Plum Tomatoes and Onion Salad

Ingredients:

- 1/2 medium red cabbage, sliced thinly
- 5 medium plum tomatoes, halved lengthwise, seeded, and thinly sliced
- 1/4 white onion, peeled, halved lengthwise, and thinly sliced
- 1 large cucumber, halved lengthwise and thinly sliced
- 5 ounces pecorino romano cheese, shredded

Dressing

- ¼ cup extra-virgin olive oil
- 2 tbsp. apple cider vinegar
- Coarse salt and black pepper

Directions:

Combine all of the dressing ingredients. Toss with the rest of the ingredients and combine well.

Red and Napa Cabbage with Cheddar Cheese Salad

Ingredients:

- 1/2 medium red cabbage, sliced thinly
- 1/2 medium Napa cabbage, sliced thinly
- 1/4 white onion, peeled, halved lengthwise, and thinly sliced
- 1 large Zucchini halved lengthwise, thinly sliced and blanched
- 3 ounces monterey jack cheese, shredded
- 3 ounces cheddar cheese, shredded

Dressing

- ¼ cup extra-virgin olive oil
- 2 splashes white wine vinegar
- Coarse salt and black pepper

Directions:

Combine all of the dressing ingredients. Toss with the rest of the ingredients and combine well.

Mangoes Peaches and Cucumber with Blue Cheese Salad

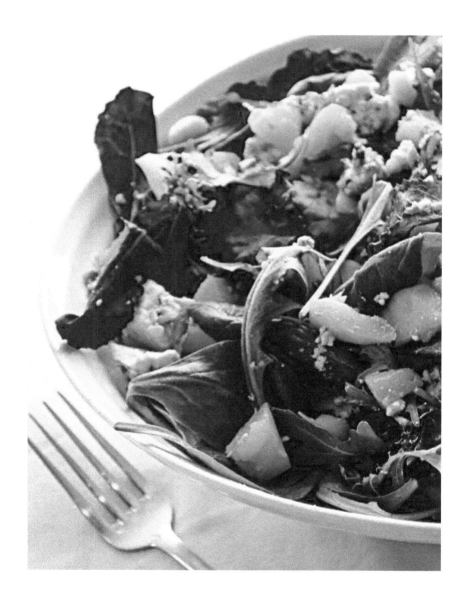

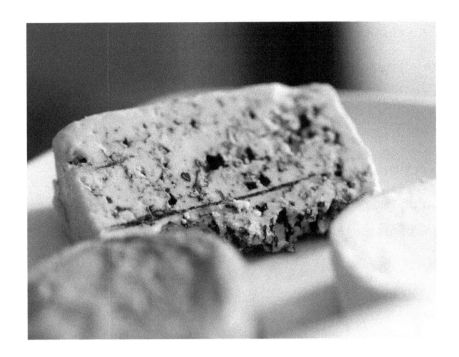

Ingredients:

- 1 cup of cubed mangoes

- 1 cup of cubed peaches

- 1/4 white onion, peeled, halved lengthwise, and thinly sliced

- 1 large cucumber, halved lengthwise and thinly sliced

Dressing

- ¼ cup extra-virgin olive oil

- 2 splashes white wine vinegar

- Coarse salt and black pepper

49

- 1 ounce blue cheese, crumbled

- 5 ounces brie cheese, crumbled

Directions:

Combine all of the dressing ingredients. Toss with the rest of the ingredients and combine well.

Kale Spinach and Cucumber with Parmesan Salad

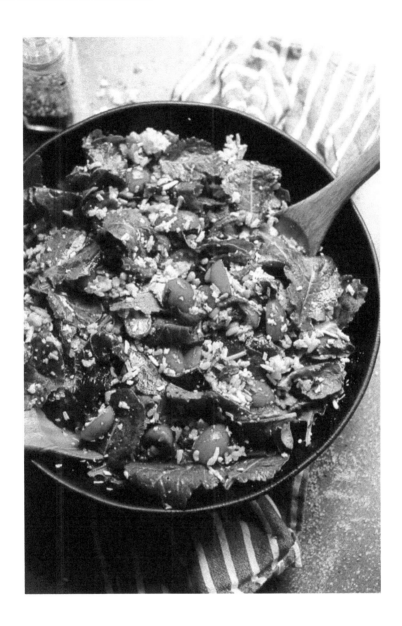

Ingredients:

- 1 bunch of kale, rinsed and drained
- 1 bunch of spinach, rinsed and drained
- 1/4 white onion, peeled, halved lengthwise, and thinly sliced
- 1 large cucumber, halved lengthwise and thinly sliced
- 2 ounces parmesan cheese, shredded
- 4 ounces ricotta cheese

Dressing

- ¼ cup extra-virgin olive oil
- 2 tbsp. apple cider vinegar
- Coarse salt and black pepper

Directions:

Combine all of the dressing ingredients. Toss with the rest of the ingredients and combine well.

Spinach Plum Tomato and Cucumber with Ricotta Cheese Salad

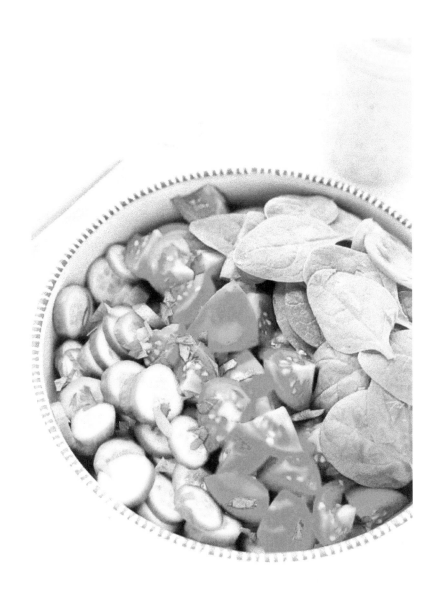

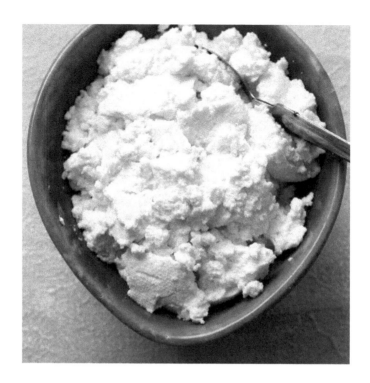

Ingredients:

- 1 bunch of watercress, rinsed and drained

- 5 medium plum tomatoes, halved lengthwise, seeded, and thinly sliced

- 1/4 white onion, peeled, halved lengthwise, and thinly sliced

- 1 large cucumber, halved lengthwise and thinly sliced

- 5 ounces ricotta cheese

Dressing

- ¼ cup extra-virgin olive oil

- 2 tbsp. apple cider vinegar

- Coarse salt and black pepper

Directions:

Combine all of the dressing ingredients. Toss with the rest of the ingredients and combine well.

Grilled Romaine Lettuce with Cream Cheese Salad

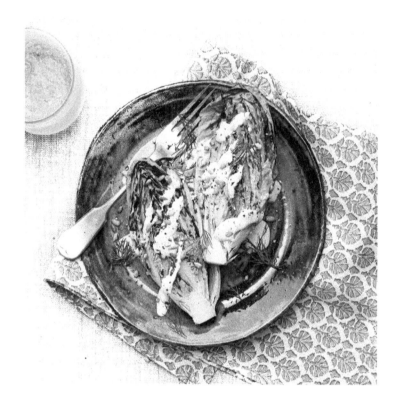

Ingredients:

- 1 head romaine lettuce, rinsed, patted and shredded

Dressing

- 2 tbsp. red wine vinegar

- 4 tablespoons extra virgin olive oil

- Freshly ground black pepper

- 5 ounces cream cheese, crumbled

- Sea salt

Grill the lettuce and/or greens over medium heat until lightly charred

Directions:

Combine all of the dressing ingredients in a food processor. Toss with the rest of the ingredients and combine well.

Grilled Boston lettuce and Gouda Cheese Salad

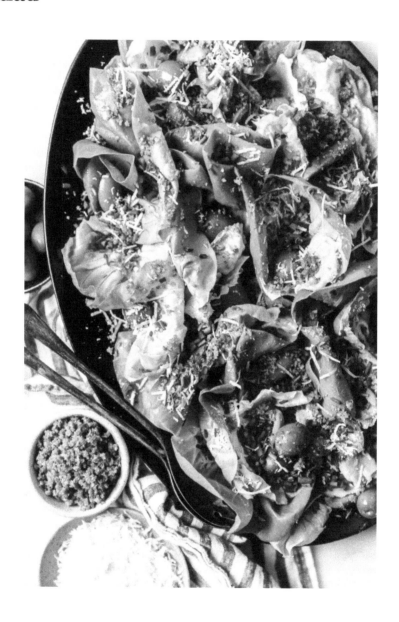

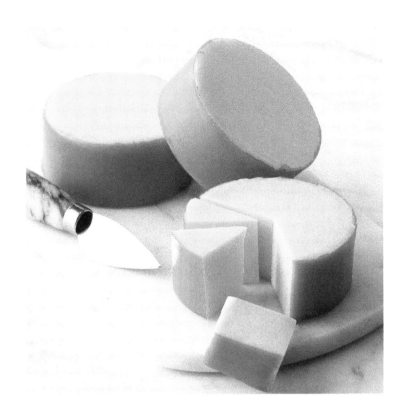

Ingredients:

- 1 head Boston lettuce, rinsed, patted and shredded

- ½ cup green olives

Dressing

- 2 tbsp. white wine vinegar

- 4 tablespoons extra virgin olive oil

- Freshly ground black pepper

- 5 ounces gouda cheese, shredded

- Sea salt

Grill the lettuce and/or greens over medium heat until lightly charred

Directions:

Combine all of the dressing ingredients in a food processor. Toss with the rest of the ingredients and combine well.

Grilled Bib Lettuce and Cream Cheese Salad

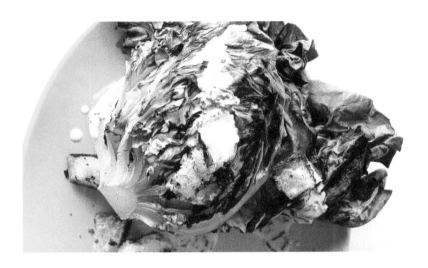

Ingredients:

- 1 head bib lettuce, rinsed, patted and shredded

- ½ cup green olives

- 5 ounces cream cheese, crumbled

Dressing

- 2 tbsp. red wine vinegar

- 4 tablespoons extra virgin olive oil

- Freshly ground black pepper

- 3/4 cup finely ground almonds

- Sea salt

Grill the lettuce and/or greens over medium heat until lightly charred

Directions:

Combine all of the dressing ingredients in a food processor. Toss with the rest of the ingredients and combine well.

Grilled Bib Lettuce and Capers Salad

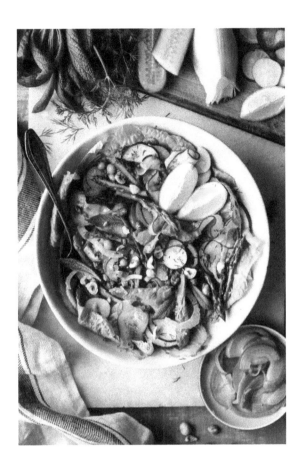

Ingredients:

- 1 head bib lettuce, rinsed, patted and shredded

- ½ cup green capers

Dressing

- 2 tbsp. white wine vinegar

- 4 tablespoons extra virgin olive oil

- Freshly ground black pepper

- 3/4 cup finely coarsely ground walnuts

- Sea salt

Grill the lettuce and/or greens over medium heat until lightly charred

Directions:

Combine all of the dressing ingredients in a food processor. Toss with the rest of the ingredients and combine well.

Grilled Bib Lettuce and Kalamata Olives Salad

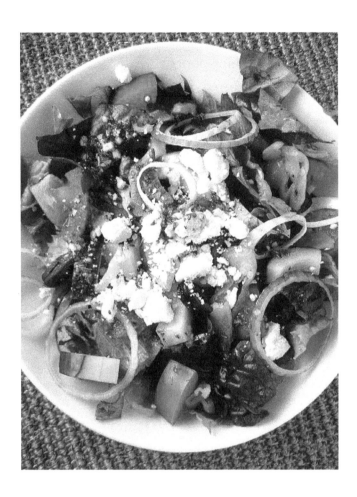

Ingredients:

- 1 head bib lettuce, rinsed, patted and shredded

- ½ cup Kalamata olives

- 5 ounces gouda cheese, shredded

Dressing

- 2 tbsp. red wine vinegar

- 4 tablespoons olive oil

- Freshly ground black pepper

- 3/4 cup finely ground almonds

- Sea salt

Grill the lettuce and/or greens over medium heat until lightly charred

Directions:

Combine all of the dressing ingredients in a food processor. Toss with the rest of the ingredients and combine well.

Romaine Lettuce Capers and Almond Vinaigrette

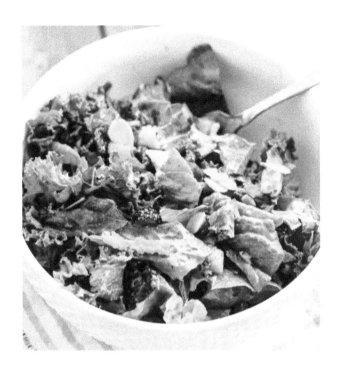

Ingredients:

- 1 head romaine lettuce, rinsed, patted and shredded

- ½ cup capers

- 5 ounces ricotta cheese

Dressing

- 2 tbsp. apple cider vinegar

- 4 tablespoons extra virgin olive oil

- Freshly ground black pepper

- 3/4 cup finely ground almonds

- Sea salt

Directions:

Combine all of the dressing ingredients in a food processor. Toss with the rest of the ingredients and combine well.

Artichoke and Artichoke Hearts with Pecorino Romano

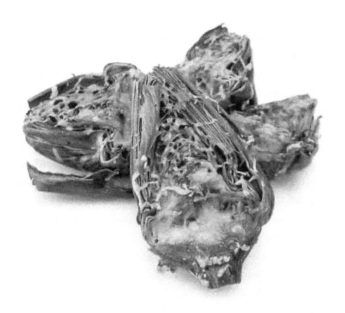

- **Ingredients:**

- 1 artichoke, rinsed & patted

- ½ cup artichoke hearts

- 5 ounces pecorino romano cheese, shredded

Dressing

- 2 tbsp. balsamic vinegar

- 4 tablespoons macadamia oil

- Freshly ground black pepper

- 3/4 cup finely ground peanuts

- Sea salt

Directions:

Combine all of the dressing ingredients in a food processor. Toss with the rest of the ingredients and combine well.

Endive with Black Olives and Artichoke Hearts

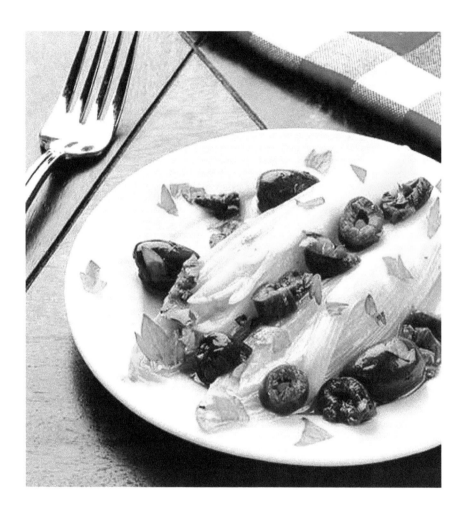

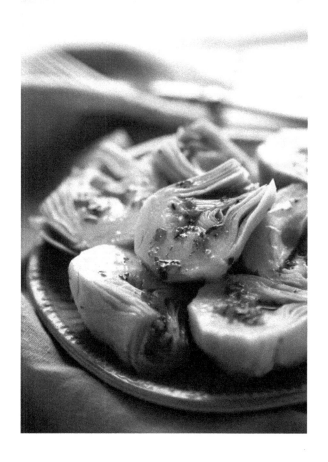

Ingredients:

- 1 head Endive, rinsed, patted and shredded

- ½ cup black olives

- ½ cup artichoke hearts

<u>Dressing</u>

- 2 tbsp. apple cider vinegar

- 4 tablespoons olive oil

- Freshly ground black pepper

- 3/4 cup finely ground almonds

- Sea salt

Directions:

Combine all of the dressing ingredients in a food processor. Toss with the rest of the ingredients and combine well.

Collard Greens Black Olive and Artichoke Heart Salad

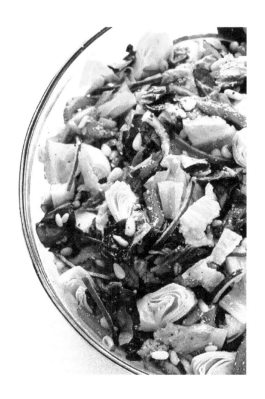

Ingredients:

- 1 bunch collard greens, rinsed, patted and shredded

- ½ cup black olives

- ½ cup artichoke hearts

Dressing

- 2 tbsp. red wine vinegar

- 4 tablespoons extra virgin olive oil

- Freshly ground black pepper

- 3/4 cup finely ground almonds

- Sea salt

Directions:

Combine all of the dressing ingredients in a food processor. Toss with the rest of the ingredients and combine well.

Bib Lettuce Black Olives and Artichoke Heart Salad

Ingredients:

- 1 head bib lettuce, rinsed, patted and shredded
- ½ cup black olives
- ½ cup artichoke hearts

Dressing

- 2 tbsp. white wine vinegar
- 4 tablespoons extra virgin olive oil
- Freshly ground black pepper
- 3/4 cup finely ground almonds
- Sea salt

Directions:

Combine all of the dressing ingredients in a food processor. Toss with the rest of the ingredients and combine well.

Romaine Lettuce with Artichoke Heart and Cashew Vinaigrette Salad

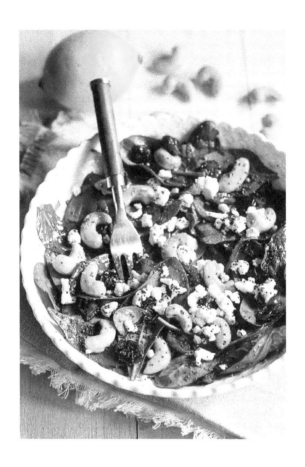

Ingredients:

- 1 head romaine lettuce, rinsed, patted and shredded

- ½ cup black olives

- ½ cup artichoke hearts

Dressing

- 2 tbsp. red wine vinegar

- 4 tablespoons olive oil

- Freshly ground black pepper

- 3/4 cup finely coarsely ground cashews

- Sea salt

Directions:

Combine all of the dressing ingredients in a food processor. Toss with the rest of the ingredients and combine well.

Beetroot Kalamata Olives and Artichoke Heart Salad

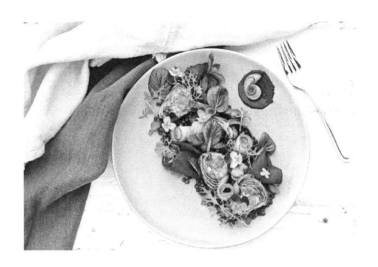

Ingredients:

- 2 beetroots, peeled and sliced lengthwise

- ½ cup Kalamata olives

- ½ cup artichoke hearts

Dressing

- 2 tbsp. white wine vinegar

- 4 tablespoons extra virgin olive oil

- Freshly ground black pepper

- 3/4 cup finely ground almonds

- Sea salt

Directions:

Combine all of the dressing ingredients in a food processor. Toss with the rest of the ingredients and combine well.

Boston Lettuce Baby Carrots and Artichoke Heart Salad

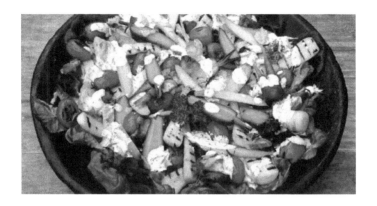

- **Ingredients:**

- 1 head Boston lettuce, rinsed, patted and shredded

- ½ cup baby carrots

- ½ cup artichoke hearts

<u>Dressing</u>

- 2 tbsp. white wine vinegar

- 4 tablespoons extra virgin olive oil

- Freshly ground black pepper

- 3/4 cup finely ground peanuts

- Sea salt

Directions:

Combine all of the dressing ingredients in a food processor. Toss with the rest of the ingredients and combine well.

Romaine Lettuce & Baby Carrots with Walnut Vinaigrette Salad

Ingredients:

- 1 bunch of kale, rinsed, patted and shredded
- ½ cup black olives
- ½ cup baby carrots

Dressing

- 2 tbsp. white wine vinegar
- 4 tablespoons extra virgin olive oil
- Freshly ground black pepper
- 3/4 cup finely coarsely ground walnuts
- Sea salt

Directions:

Combine all of the dressing ingredients in a food processor. Toss with the rest of the ingredients and combine well.

Romaine Lettuce Green Olives and Artichoke Heart with Macadamia Vinaigrette

Ingredients:

- 1 head Boston lettuce, rinsed, patted and shredded
- ½ cup green olives
- ½ cup artichoke hearts

Dressing

- 2 tbsp. balsamic vinegar
- 4 tablespoons macadamia oil
- Freshly ground black pepper
- 3/4 cup finely coarsely ground cashews
- Sea salt

Directions:

Combine all of the dressing ingredients in a food processor. Toss with the rest of the ingredients and combine well.

Collard Greens with Baby Corn Salad

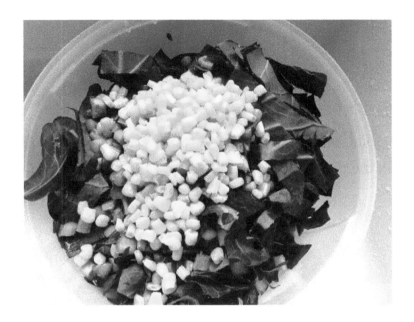

Ingredients:

- 1 bunch of collard greens

- ½ cup black olives

- ½ cup canned baby corn

Dressing

- 2 tbsp. red wine vinegar

- 4 tablespoons extra virgin olive oil

- Freshly ground black pepper

- 3/4 cup finely ground almonds

- Sea salt

Directions:

Combine all of the dressing ingredients in a food processor. Toss with the rest of the ingredients and combine well.

Bib Lettuce Black Olives and Baby Corn with Almond Vinaigrette Salad

Ingredients:

- 1 head Bib lettuce, rinsed, patted and shredded
- ½ cup black olives
- ½ cup canned baby corn

Dressing

- 2 tbsp. white wine vinegar
- 4 tablespoons olive oil
- Freshly ground black pepper
- 3/4 cup finely ground almonds
- Sea salt

Directions:

Combine all of the dressing ingredients in a food processor. Toss with the rest of the ingredients and combine well.

Mixed Greens Olives and Artichoke Heart Salad

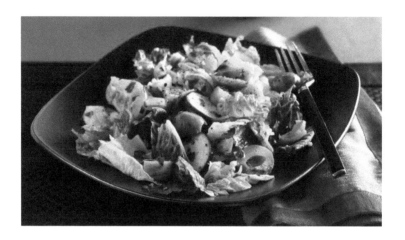

Ingredients:

- 1 bunch of mixed greens, rinsed, patted and shredded

- ½ cup black olives

- ½ cup artichoke hearts

Dressing

- 2 tbsp. white wine vinegar

- 4 tablespoons extra virgin olive oil

- Freshly ground black pepper

- 3/4 cup finely coarsely ground walnuts

- Sea salt

Directions:

Combine all of the dressing ingredients in a food processor. Toss with the rest of the ingredients and combine well.

Artichoke Capers and Artichoke Heart Salad

Ingredients:

- 1 artichoke, rinsed, patted and shredded
- ½ cup capers
- ½ cup artichoke hearts

Dressing

- 2 tbsp. white wine vinegar
- 4 tablespoons extra virgin olive oil
- Freshly ground black pepper
- 3/4 cup finely ground almonds
- Sea salt

Directions:

Combine all of the dressing ingredients in a food processor. Toss with the rest of the ingredients and combine well.

Bib Lettuce with Tomatillo Dressing

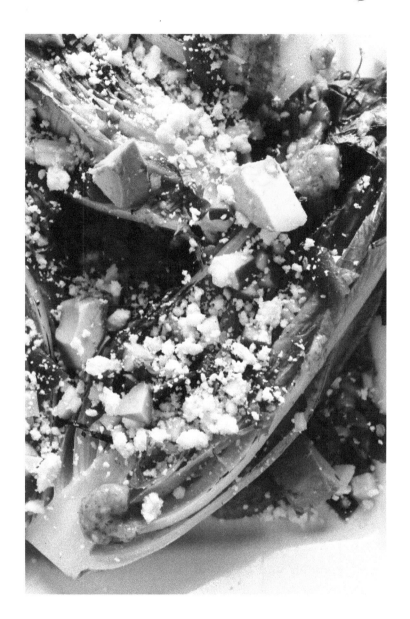

Ingredients:

- 1 head Bib lettuce, shredded
- 4 large tomatoes, seeded and chopped
- 4 radishes, thinly sliced

Dressing

- 6 tomatillos, rinsed and halved
- 1 jalapeno, halved
- 1 white onion, quartered
  2 tablespoons extra virgin olive oil
- Kosher salt and freshly ground black pepper
- 1/2 teaspoon ground cumin
- 1 cup Dairy free cream cheese
- 2 tablespoons fresh lemon juice

Directions:

Preheat the oven to 400 degrees F. For the dressing, place the tomatillos, jalapeno and onion on a cookie sheet. Drizzle with olive oil and sprinkle with salt and pepper. Roast in the oven for 25- 30 min. until vegetables begin to brown and slightly darken.

Transfer to a food processor and let it cool then blend. Add the rest of the ingredients and refrigerate for an hour. Toss with the rest of the ingredients and combine well.

Plum Tomato Cucumber and Ricotta Salad

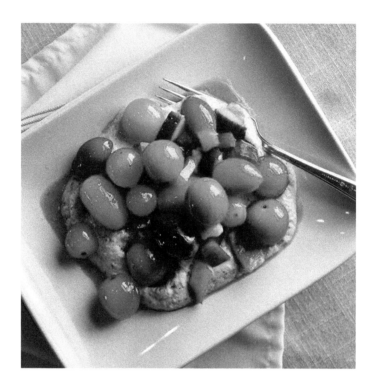

Ingredients:

- 5 medium plum tomatoes, halved lengthwise, seeded, and thinly sliced

- 1/4 white onion, peeled, halved lengthwise, and thinly sliced

- 1 large cucumber, halved lengthwise and thinly sliced

- 5 ounces ricotta cheese

Dressing

- ¼ cup extra-virgin olive oil

- 2 splashes white wine vinegar

- Coarse salt and black pepper

Directions:

Combine all of the dressing ingredients. Toss with the rest of the ingredients and combine well.

Tomato and Zucchini Salad

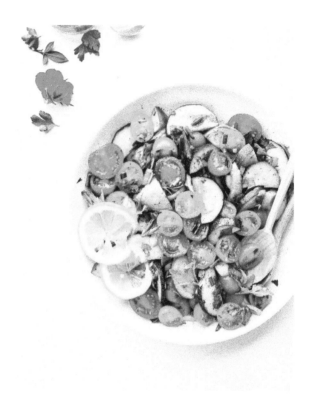

Ingredients:

- 5 medium tomatoes, halved lengthwise, seeded, and thinly sliced

- 1/4 white onion, peeled, halved lengthwise, and thinly sliced

- 1 large Zucchini halved lengthwise ,thinly sliced & blanched

- 5 ounces mozarella cheese, shredded

Dressing

- ¼ cup extra-virgin olive oil

- 2 tbsp. apple cider vinegar

- Coarse salt and black pepper

Directions:

Combine all of the dressing ingredients. Toss with the rest of the ingredients and combine well.

Plum Tomato and Onion Salad

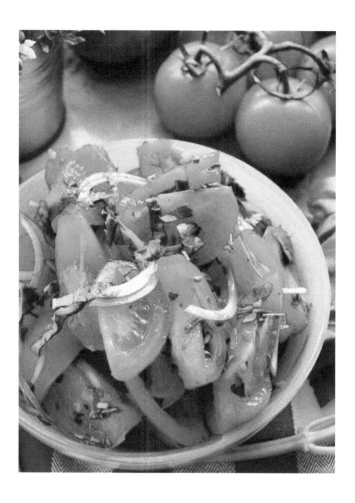

Ingredients:

- 5 medium plum tomatoes, halved lengthwise, seeded, and thinly sliced

- 1/4 white onion, peeled, halved lengthwise, and thinly sliced

- 1 large cucumber, halved lengthwise and thinly sliced

<u>Dressing</u>

- ¼ cup extra-virgin olive oil

- 2 tbsp. apple cider vinegar

- Coarse salt and black pepper

<u>Prep</u>

Directions:

Combine all of the dressing ingredients. Toss with the rest of the ingredients and combine well.

Heirloom Tomato Salad

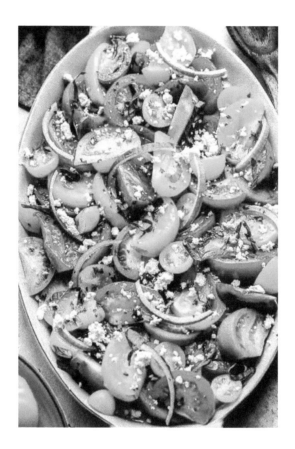

Ingredients:

- 3 Heirloom tomatoes, halved lengthwise, seeded, and thinly sliced

- 1/4 white onion, peeled, halved lengthwise, and thinly sliced

- 1 large cucumber, halved lengthwise and thinly sliced

<u>Dressing</u>

- ¼ cup extra-virgin olive oil

- 2 splashes white wine vinegar

- Coarse salt and black pepper

Directions:

Combine all of the dressing ingredients. Toss with the rest of the ingredients and combine well.

Artichoke Heart and Plum Tomato Salad

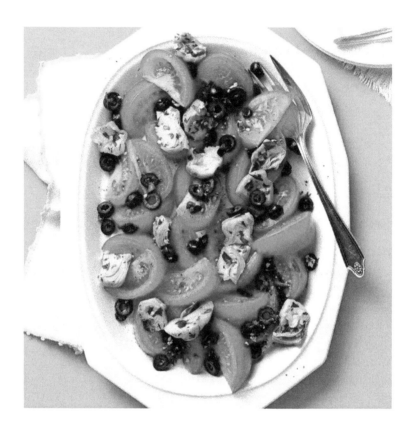

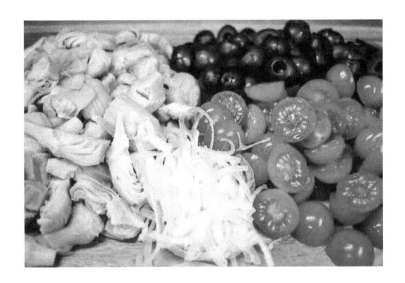

Ingredients:

- 6 Artichoke Hearts (Canned)

- 5 medium plum tomatoes, halved lengthwise, seeded, and thinly sliced

- 1/4 white onion, peeled, halved lengthwise, and thinly sliced

- 1 large cucumber, halved lengthwise and thinly sliced

Dressing

- ¼ cup extra-virgin olive oil

- 2 splashes white wine vinegar

- Coarse salt and black pepper

Directions:

Combine all of the dressing ingredients. Toss with the rest of the ingredients and combine well.

Mixed Greens Feta Cheese and Tomato Salad

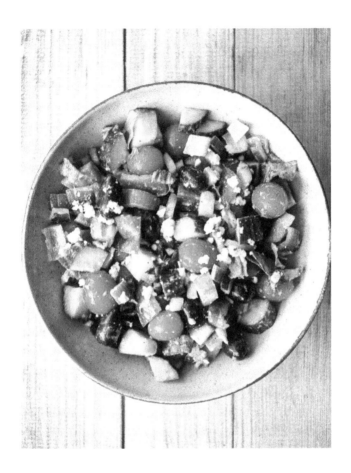

Ingredients:

- 1 bunch Meslcun, rinsed and drained

- 5 medium tomatoes, halved lengthwise, seeded, and thinly sliced

- 1/4 white onion, peeled, halved lengthwise, and thinly sliced

- 1 large cucumber, halved lengthwise and thinly sliced

- 5 ounces feta cheese, crumbled

Dressing

- ¼ cup extra-virgin olive oil

- 2 tbsp. apple cider vinegar

- Coarse salt and black pepper

Directions:

Combine all of the dressing ingredients. Toss with the rest of the ingredients and combine well.

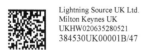

Lightning Source UK Ltd.
Milton Keynes UK
UKHW020635280521
384530UK00001B/47

9 781802 695786